©2018

Ahia True Peace
zunyaz@zoho.com

All Rights Reserved.

ISBN-13: 978-1726420259

ISBN-10: 1726420256

CHANDRA MUDRA

AHIA TRUE PEACE

Prativijanati Agastya and Lopamudra
Thanks Love for all the loving support and for taking the pictures!

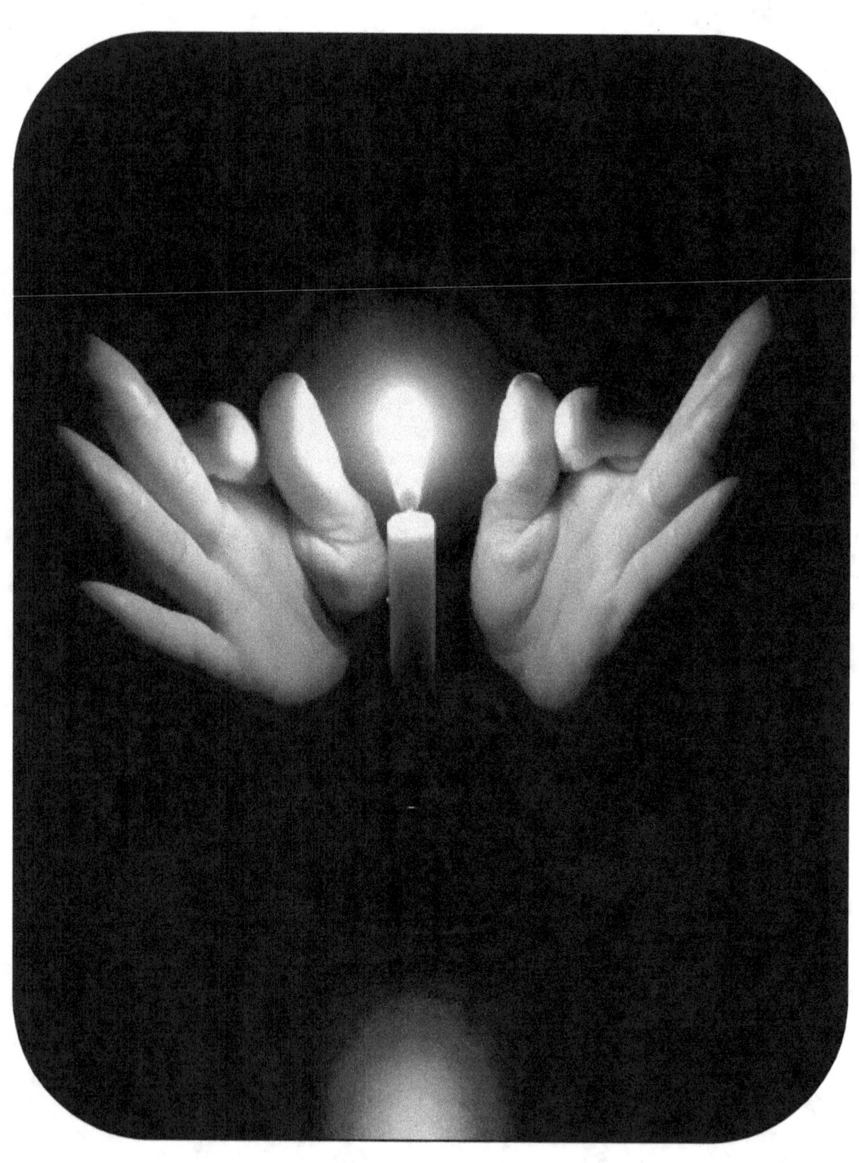

Shiva Mudra (Jnana)
The Release of All Ignorance

The Meaning Behind Chandra Mudra

This book was named in honor of the moon. Chandra translates into 'luminous.' The mudra in this book can bring illumination to your changing seasons, if you want it to.

The Moon plays a pivotal role in Vedic Astrology Jyotish. Jyotish means the movement of light within the Cosmos. Some might say that Western Astrology is Solar based whereas Jyotish is Lunar based and therefore, better attuned to the Feminine Aspect of Creation.

Chandra watches us, nurtures us and holds us during the dark night. She regulates the seasons, tides, cycles of Earth and so does she for the rest of us.

The Moon is also in the AUM (OM) symbol as the dividing conscious between the Unchanging Eternal and the rest of Creation. It is the crescent shape underneath the diamond.

Some call this plane of consciousness Maya. Others recognize it where the unified Spark of Creation occurs, where everything is divided aka created.

Whatever way you look at it, it's the last gate one must past until one enters the Realm Beyond Realms.

To help you ride the wave of energy as it passes, to keep pace with all the astrological influences there is in the Universe, to bring your life to balance when you swing out of place, that is what mudra is for.

If you already have a yoga practice or are just started one, mudra will accompany beautifully and give new dimension. Speaking from personal experience, I have been blessed greatly by it.

Honor Chandra, honor the passing tides in your internal and external realms, as you do so, you naturally return to cosmic alignment.

Mudra Yoga is just another way in which to do all that, simply and effectively.

Namaste.
the silence within me witnesses the silence within you

Introduction to Mudra • What Mudra Is • How to Do Mudra
Simple Suggestions • Things To Know
Sanatana Dharma, Silence, Intention, Surrender, Peace

FOUNDATIONAL MUDRA

Introduction
To Mudra

What Mudra Is

Mudra has been done since humans developed hands. In India and other cultures, it has been understood for millennia how the hands have power and what they can do, simply with intention and focus.

Mudra is a Sanskrit word that means 'to lock.' As you position your hands and fingers in a certain way, keeping them steady and locked, so do you also lock your field into a certain type of energy flow.

Perhaps you have seen a Tai Chi push someone over from a distance, just by pushing their hands in the air? Or maybe you have seen another type of master break wood or brick with their bare hands. The mechanics are the same.

But instead of effecting other things and people outside of us thru hand movements and energy cultivation, we mudra to rearrange and enhance the qualities of our own inner world.

When you mudra, you connect to a very ancient, time tested way of relating to yourself, your body and the eternal consciousness. Your Ancestors have done it and now you get to reap the benefits as well.

Every mudra is a prayer to experience the release of all thoughts and feelings of separation and experience the blossoming of ecstasy that naturally arises when you unify your consciousness into one light stream.

It is known in Traditional Chinese medicine that the hand is connected to every other part of the body. So when you move your hands in a certain way, you also affect the well-being of the rest of your body and ultimately, the purity of your consciousness.

Here's to a clear mind and pure heart!

How Mudra Works

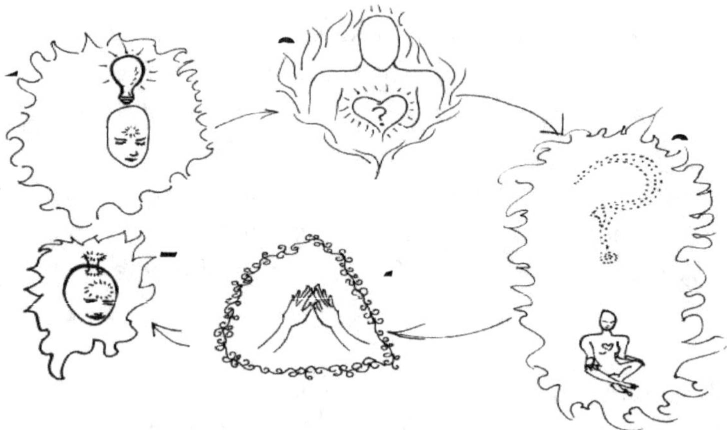

1.   You are having an experience where you feel out of balance or in lack. You then come to realize what you are lacking and what you need in that moment.

2.   You wonder how to embody what you are lacking.

3.   The Universe hears your question and begins to formulate the vibrations you are missing.

4.   You form the mudra with your hands which become like an antenna for the vibrations the Universe has formulated.

5.   Embodying the vibrations feels good! You field spins up in a new way, receiving the new energy from the Universe.

Mudra yoga is an exercise is motion, the change in perspective until we come to a place where there can be no more change. The eternal self is forever changeless. Mudra is about sustaining the focus, the power, the wisdom and the natural way within us. Reaffirming our place as conscious stewards. It is complementary to any other practice you could be doing.

Arms and hands are the extensions of the heart, so is the voice. What are the heart and voice an extension of? The eternal self.

Have you ever wondered, where exactly your voice comes from? Beyond the vocal chords, beyond that. It is the same place everything comes from. This place is infinite and limitless.

The body is a temple, the body is also a sacred instrument, the container of this limitless energy. Use it wisely.

How To Mudra

In essence, there is no wrong way really but, with precision, there can be more precise results.

Look thru the list of mudra and notice the ones that jump out at you. The ones you resonate with now will change over time. If you know exactly what you need assistance with, you might look for a mudra based on what is happening in your life.

Take special notice of how the fingers connect, either thru the absolute tips of the fingers or the pads. Find your place. Everyone's hands are different so everyone has their own 'sweet spot.' You can reverse hands too, it doesn't matter which hand is on top, the right or left.

Adjust and readjust as you will to find t and once you do, you will be able to feel it. It will feel easy, like gears just sunk into place, not like you are forcing your fingers into position. It's like there is a subtle magnetism pulling your fingers together, keeping them in that spot.

Silence your mind but open your intuition channels. Be open to hearing, feeling and seeing in your mind's eye whatever comes up. Making sure your body feels comfortable and your consciousness feel safe is a key part. Whatever you do, don't resist, just sink in!

You can do mudra whenever, in the morning upon rising before getting out of bed, when eating, when waiting in line, during meditation, during a test, at a rave, in the middle of a movie. You pick the place and length of time that works best for you.

That's sanatana dharma.

You pick to hold the mudra for however long feels best. If you still aren't sure, 15 minutes is a good place to start. Once you have found your positioning, you can move your hands around to different places. You can hold the mudra against different parts of your body, on the ground, in the sky.

Remember, whatever feels best!

Setting aside some time to relax and meditate might make the experience more interactive for you if you are just a beginner, as for as feeling energy goes.

Incense, candles, gentle music, low lighting and being next to a river or in the woods can also help you open up and receive. You can turn this time into an extra special time, into a ritual or ceremony if you are so inclined.

Simple Suggestions

Here are some suggestions to add to your mudra ritual.

First wash your hands and dry them completely. Then, anoint your hands with special anointing fluid, along with your 3rd eye, in the middle of your forehead. This will help you open your receptive, intuitive centers.

Feel free to improvise the recipes, you might have some other ideas.

Sanatana dharma!

Hand Wash Recipe

- *Purified Water*
- *Himalayan (or similar, unrefined, natural) Salt*
- *Flower Essence or Flower Hydrosol such as Jasmine, Rose*

Use a big bowl, pour in water, gently mix in salt. Let hands air dry, slowly.

The salt clears the energy in your hands and the flower consciousness brings sweetness to your energy field.

Hand Anointing Recipe

- *Unrefined, organic oil or butter of any kind – coconut, apricot, jojoba oil or cocoa, shea butter suggested*
- *Colloidal silver*
- *Lavender and Citrus essential oils (or any of your favorites)*

Mix all ingredients well in a container that is easy to open and pour or with a wide lid if you used butter.

Cover your hands completely from your wrists up, on both sides, like a prayer in action. Now you are ready to go!

Things
To Know

Before jumping right in, let's take some time to understand a few things, at least, mentally before, at most, bodily embodiment.

Sanatana Dharma

I'm sure you have heard the word 'Hindu' or 'Hinduism.' Hindu is an outsider's name for something, looking in. Just like Native tribes have been renamed by conquering outsiders and given new names, the same can be said for Hinduism. The name 'Hindu' was given to the people who lived near the Indus River.

Originally, Hinduism was Sanatana Dharma. In reality, Hinduism is Sanatana Dharma and will always be Sanatana Dharma. Sanatana Dharma can never change or go away. Sanatana Dharma, directly translated, means the eternal law. I translate it into 'natural cosmic order.'

Basically it says that the Universe and Cosmos have a natural order, law or way. If you follow that order within yourself, your life will flourish as you will. If you go against the natural law and your inner guidance, then your life will constantly be filled with strife, pain, anguish and sorrow. Follow the natural flow and grow, go against the natural flow and resist and you will pay dearly. As aspects of the ultimate Creator in human form, we always have a choice.

Sanatana Dharma means that you do whatever you want to reach
Godhead, given that you don't overly harm another on the way to
get there, that is against the natural world order because humanity's
natural way of being is genuinely collaborative and supportive of
everyone else's journey.

Sanatana Dharma is you witnessing the separation within yourself
and then proceeding to do whatever you damn well please in order
to get that feeling of separation from All That Is to cease and to then
realize One with the One, your Self, your eternal Self, within.
It is in the degrees and concepts of separation from your Self where
all pain arises, even when those experiences of pain include other
people. They are still You, just in perceived other forms.

Continuously reach for the One, the Eternal Self and do whatever
floats your boat in the meantime. Just as long as it feels good,
eventually, everything will be great.

Silence

Deep silence is key to knowing the eternal self. Experiencing bliss,
letting go of self-doubt. In order to get there, our entire
consciousness, mind and body must be undistracted, clearly
attuned, deftly defined and least resistant.

Silence the mind sounds like forcing. Some of us were told to be
silent in school, silent at the table, silent in the store, silent at home,
but this is a different type of silence.

This is a silence that drowns out everything in the world. This
silence brings a peace so wide so deep, it goes on forever. Beyond
words, beyond thoughts, beyond feelings, beyond anything you can
think of.

In order to get there, you may have to go thru some very unsilent thoughts, feelings, repressed and forgotten. That is OK. It is all a part of the process. Cutting out media helps.

The deep silence helps the mudra flow.

Ultimately, you will reach a point of the silence of the guru. Don't try to hard, don't try to force anything. Just sit back, relax, let go and sink. Just let it happen.

Intention

What exactly is intention? It's when the physical and energetic realms perfectly align. We carry out the action in the energetic realms and the physical realms.

We have intentions to have different experiences. You intended to read this book and look, now you are! Intentions can include anything your heart desires, anything in the physical to manifesting clarity or openness in our internal realms.

When we intend, magic happens. The stars realign, the Universe shifts. That is the glory of being Creators in human bodies at this time. We have the manifestational abilities. Put that gift to good use! Don't waste it! You have it for good reason!

Now go to work!

Surrender

Surrender is so important if we want to create and experience life on a really deep level. Until you realize all wars arise through your own self, and that all battles are only with yourself, then you will be running in circles, constantly trying to put out fires.

Non judgmental, open to receive whatever comes, in whatever form it arrives. Like welcoming a guest into your house who has just knocked upon your door and has a bunch of presents they've been hanging on to in hopes to pass onto you one day.

Lay down your sword!

Peace

Peace comes as you know exactly who and what you really are, fully. With surrender, comes deep peace finally, naturally, not strained. And inside yourself, a domino effect is started.

Surrender leads to peace. Peace leads to love. Peace leads to an open, uninhibited heart and clear mind. A mind that is free and clear leads to the chance and ability to listen to your clear inner voice and experience your clear inner vision.

Peace is the foundation intimate relationship with our home Earth and all her kingdoms and all of Creation.

Ultimately, peace can only lead to more peace!

REMEMBER

Find your own rhythm.

Inner movement leads to clarity of sound, feeling, thought and
peace.

Feel out the mudra, find your own resting place!

And above all else…

Have Fun Already!!!

FOUNDATIONAL MUDRA

Stairway to Heaven
Warmups

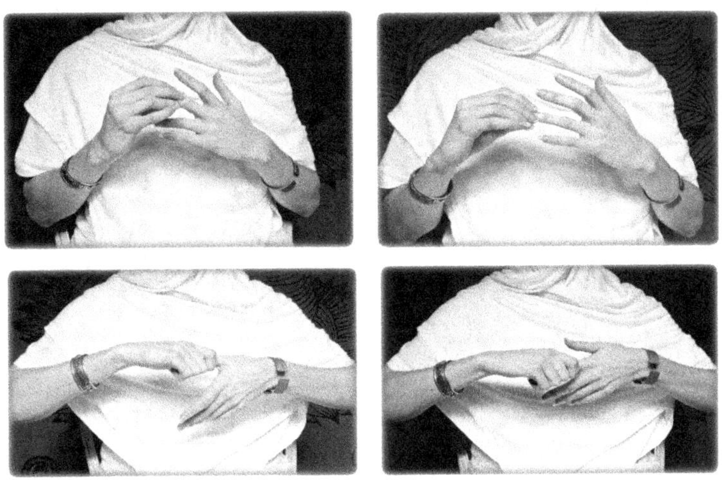

Massage each finger, moving up and unto the next. Then pulling on each finger from different knuckles.

Moving like a circular stairway.

This helps the energy move more freely before doing other mudra.

It's also nice just on it's own to stimulate every system, as your hands connect to every other part of your body.

Ignition

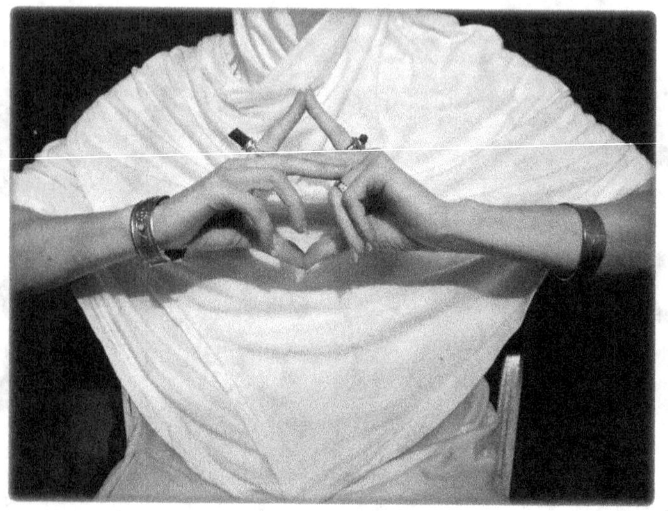

1st Finger to 1st Finger, Thumb to Thumb, Middle Finger inside
finger crease

This mudra is done with the intention to repattern your energy and body, 'now it's mudra time, time to relax, sink in and feel deep!'

This is about getting your energy bodies ready to accept the energy movements about to be bestowed upon you and will give you time to settle into this new rhythm.

This mudra is also good to do when beginning new creative projects or even, just starting the day!

Surrender

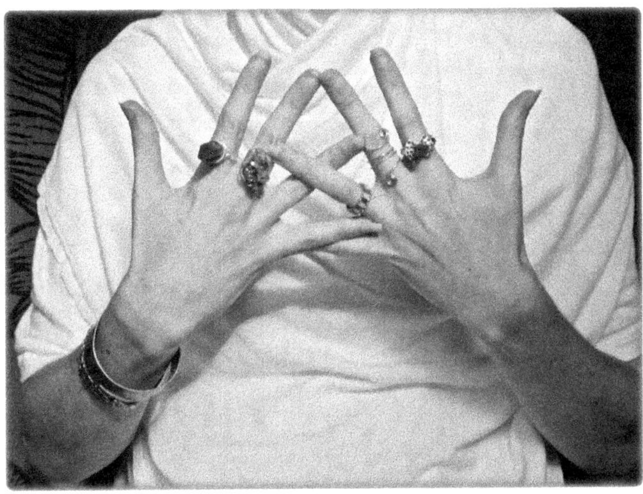

3rd Fingertips to 2nd Finger Knuckles, 4th Finger to Inside Crease

Surrender is perhaps the most daunting yet the most pivotal thing you can do in your life.

This is not necessarily surrender towards another human, but surrender to the ultimate divine flow of creation. To the eternal self.

To become a devotee of you. And then to live a life with surrender as your foundation. Tied into non-violence and adhimsa, which is also a Sanskrit word that means non-harm.

Surrender is the same as ho'oponopono.

Ho'oponopono is a Hawaiian word that means ' to make right.' It is the act of laying to rest all past transgresses in your ancestral family line.

Structure

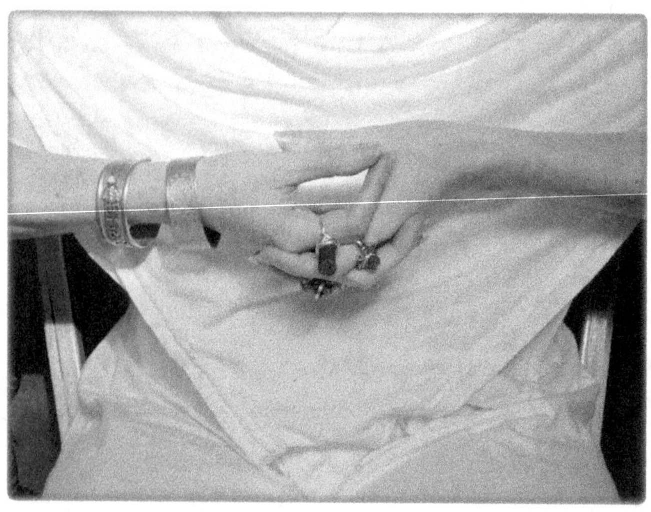

Thumb to 1st fingerpads, fingers interlocked

This mudra has to do with the format of structure and the very makeup of your creation on the elemental and DNA level. It is true your body is your highest temple.

This is a good mudra for the body and to heal any health issues you may be having. If you have forgotten what it means to be home, that your body is home.

This is not some dogmatic platitude, it is the greatest blessing to realize home is the truth of your being as a multifaceted expression of the eternal self.

Make peace with the earth element.

Natural Power

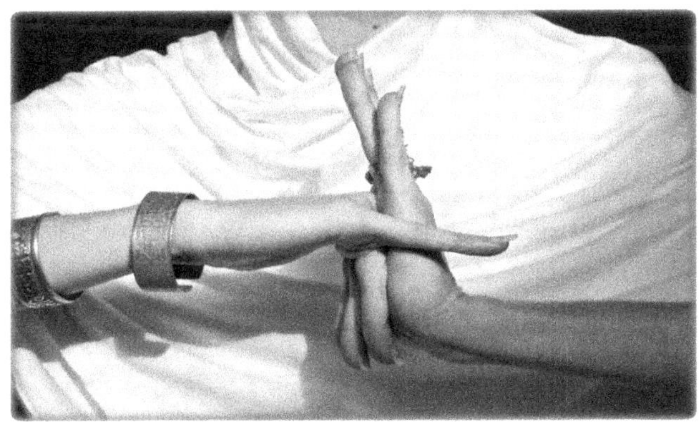

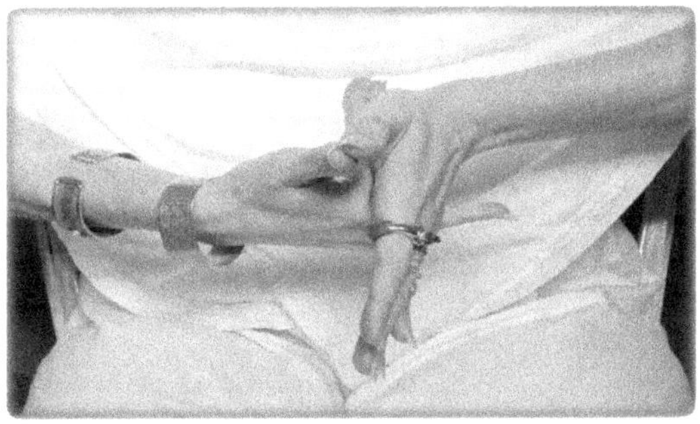

Power that comes from neither above or below, this power is self-evident. Based in the natural world order or the way of sanatana dharma. Rooted in awareness of both the individual and the group, this power is all pervasive, dependent on nothing other than the potent expression of itself.

Some might call this shakti.

Breath of Life

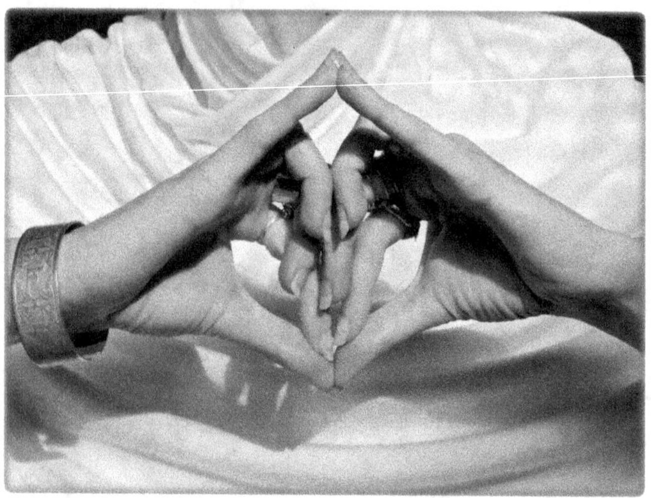

1st, 2nd, 3rd Finger Knuckles Touch 1st Finger Touches Thumb

Breath of life is associated with creativity of expression. The soft unfoldment. Understanding cycles of creation and destruction, the in-breath and the out-breath.

To go back to the beginning, to the source of all creations, therefore implying the possibility of all time space and form awaiting your direction.

This is a good mudra to clarify your inner channels of presence and expression, to get your creative juices flowing.

All Encompassing Love

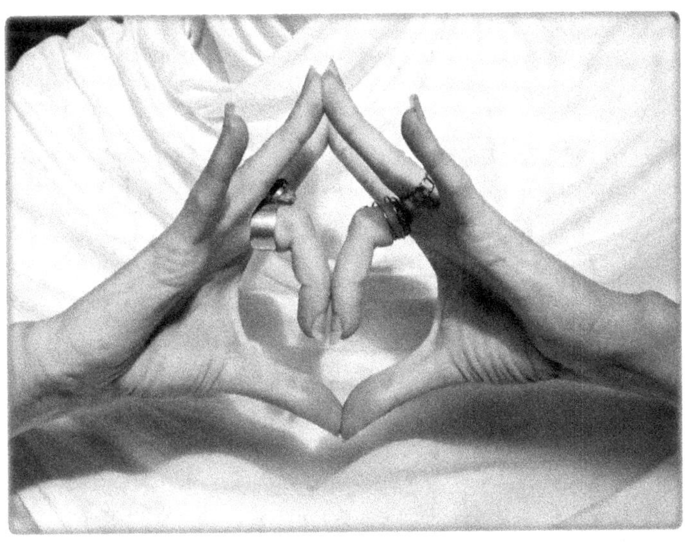

2st Finger Knuckles Touch

All compassionate is the way of the eternal self. Compassion is the embracement of everyone and every event you experience and see experienced around you, in acceptance and gentle love, without the need to force change or stagnation. Holding in contentment until all aspects realize the same thing – that there is no separation and all is of the eternal self, never separated, never once, never will.

Do you put conditions on your love? You love one thing or person more than another when in truth, all are equal expressions of the same thing, the same eternal expression. Do you want to be free from the bondage of overt judgment that is harsh in lieu of a level headed discernment that allows your love to flow freely unto all creations, including yourself?

Then this is the perfect mudra to allow that to come to fruition.

Moksha

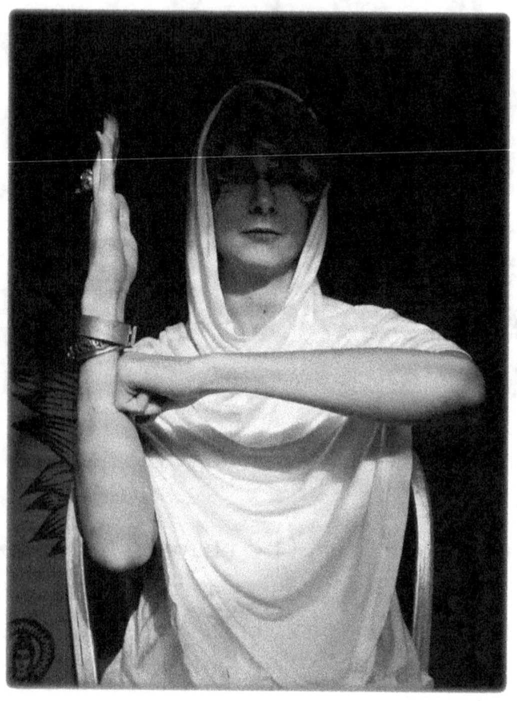

Moksha is the Sanskrit word for in other words, freedom. True freedom is the release of the thoughtform of karma, living for today, in light of what has happened in the past and what could happen in the future.

What is true freedom to you? How deep does it run?

Divine Union

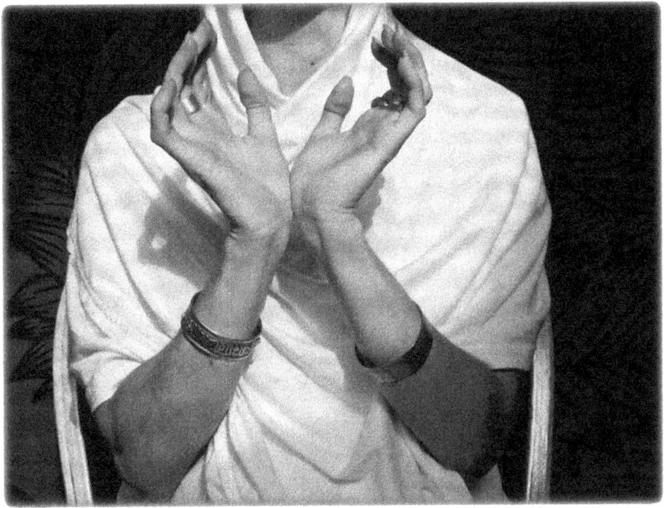

Corner of Hands Touch

Divine Union is the union of body, soul, mind, heart within and of yourself and then the union of yourself with the creational realm in which you live, including all other aspects of that.

The union of male and female.

A good mudra to do if you are feeling like there is 'something missing' or if you feel as though you are separate from either your internal masculine or feminine expression within..

Umoga

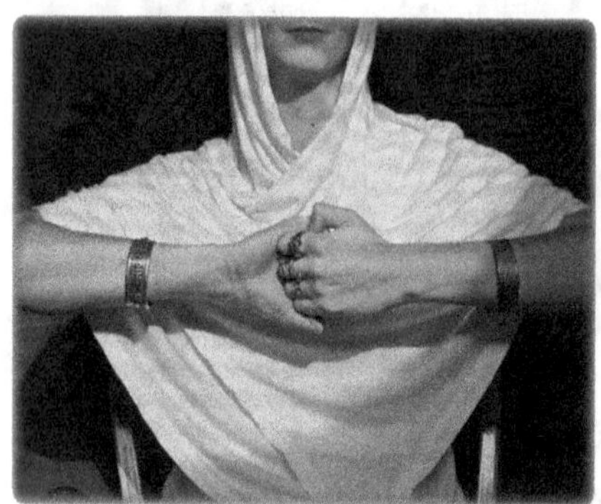 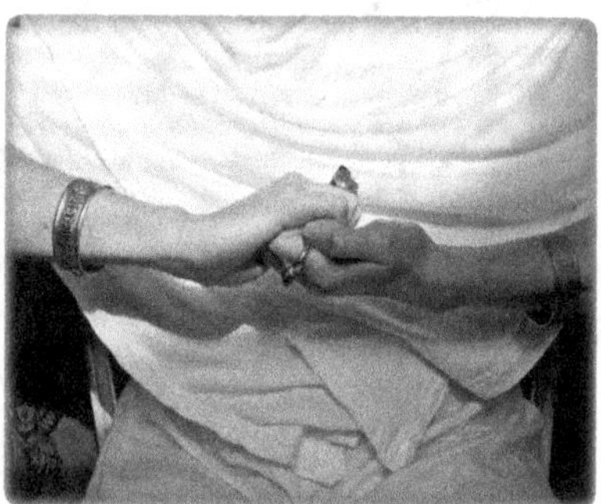

1st thru 4th Finger Wrap Thumbs go into wrapped hands

Umoga is an African word for 'unity.'

Divine Union expressed in a group setting. Finding the natural rhythm and balance with Earth and all her kingdoms, along with other humans within the spin of the Universe.

Where everyone in the group is realigned to the natural world order, harmony is assured.

Natural Leadership

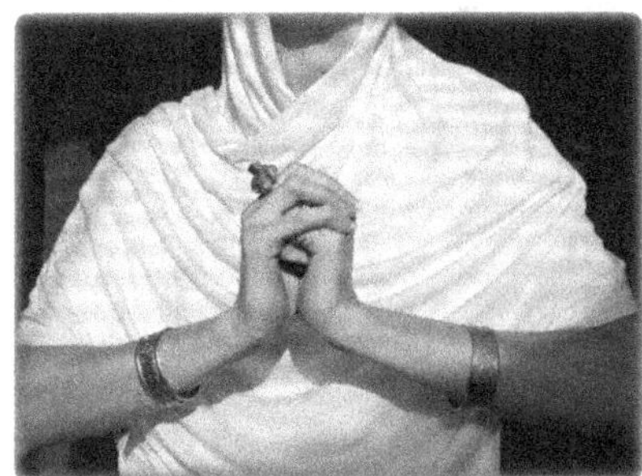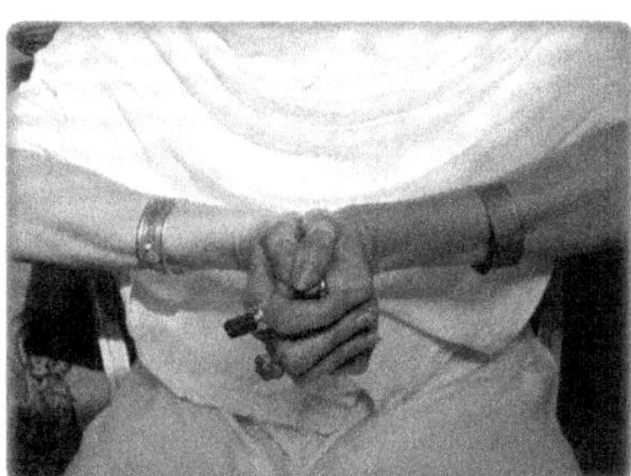

Inside Fingers curled, Top Thumb holding down inside Thumb

Are you the leader of yourself? Have you heard the call yet? Do you wish to let go all notions of being a slave, being less than, being directed by materialistic gains and limited mind think?

Being a natural leader means self-appointed and self-directed. Being a natural leader means sometimes stepping out where few dare to tread. Being a natural leader sometimes means retreating in situations where others are rushing to be first in line, depends on the place and time.

In either situation, the leader within you reigns and you do what you deem is right.

If you are needing a clear inner director that takes charge and knows what to do in harmony with natural world order, your own personal sanatana dharma, then this mudra is perfect.

Boundaries

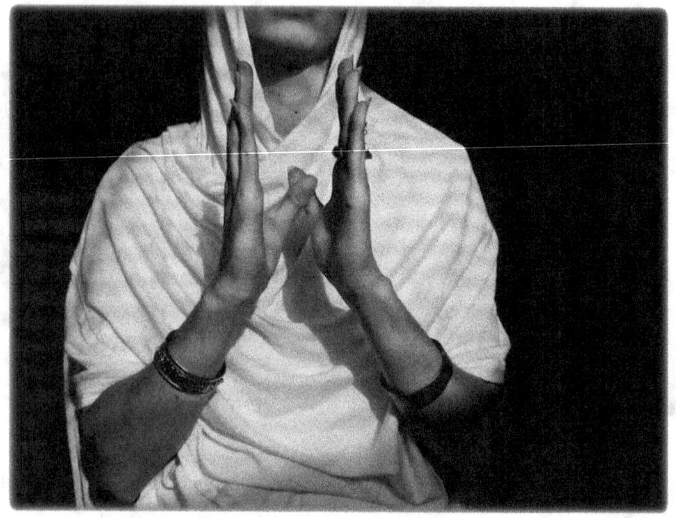

Thumbs Touch

Sometimes we must create boundaries in our life to heal. Like the body separates a tumor from the rest of the body to preserve the heal of the entire system, so too we need to cut certain people, thinking patterns and behaviors out of live to come into balance again.

If you've been walked on too many times and been someone's rug, this is a great mudra to do to remember how to create sacred space and claim your space, your body, mind and life as your own, aside from harm.

Hope

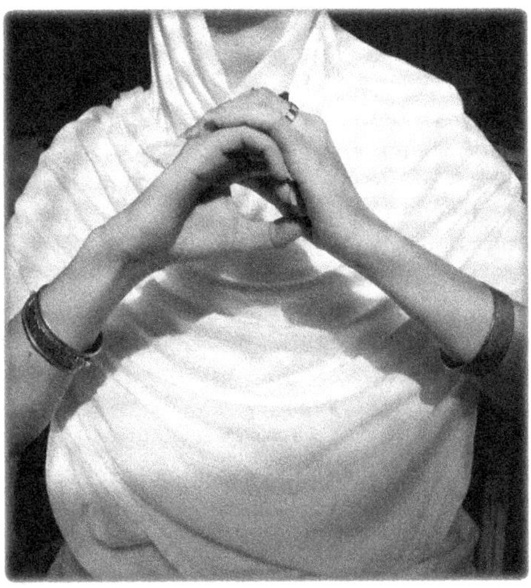

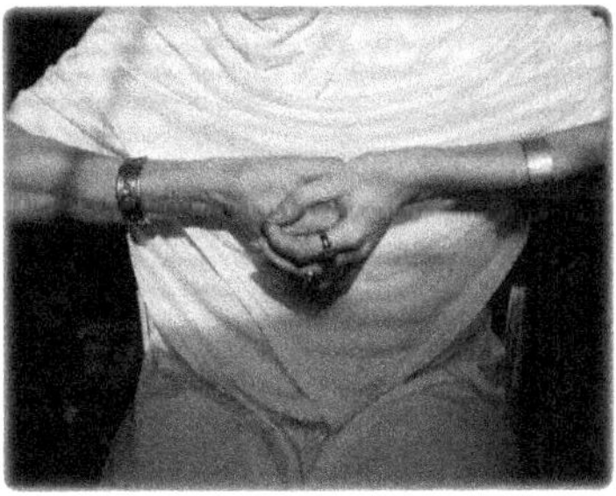

Thumb and 1st fingertip touch

When there is no end in sight, the light at the end of the tunnel. Release all density and heavy feelings along with the belief that nothing can change.

Everything changes.

Abundance

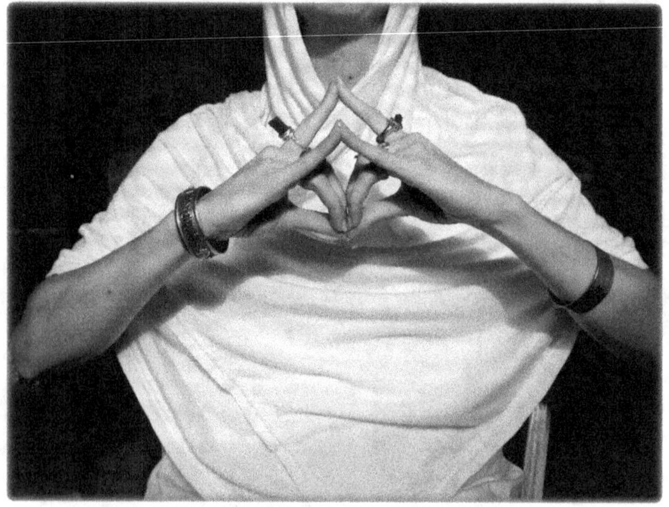

2nd and 3rd Finger Touching Thumb

Abundance is not just what you have in the physical, it is a state of awareness. Understanding you are the Source means there is no limitations.

Embrace an abundant state of mind and experiences in your life will follow.

Magnitude

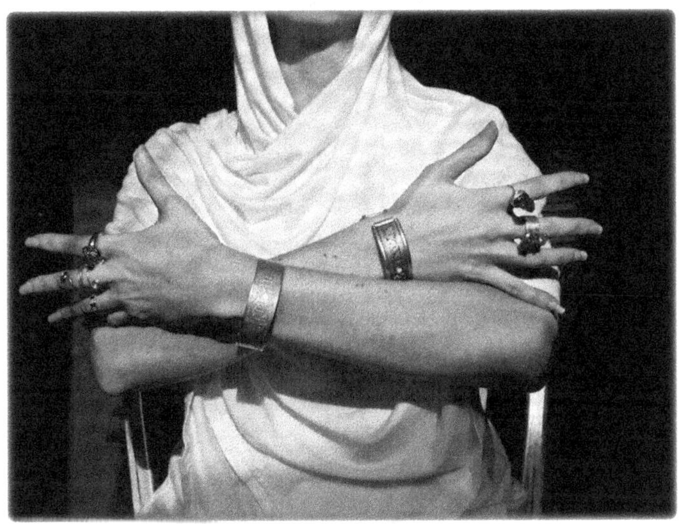

All Fingers Spread, Pinky laid on Arm

The expanded view of things. Releasing concepts of limitation. See the big picture. Realize your interconnectedness with all of creation.

You are boundless!

Stealth

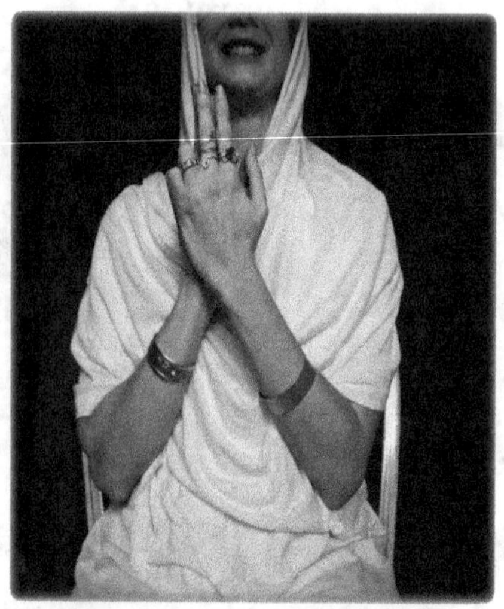

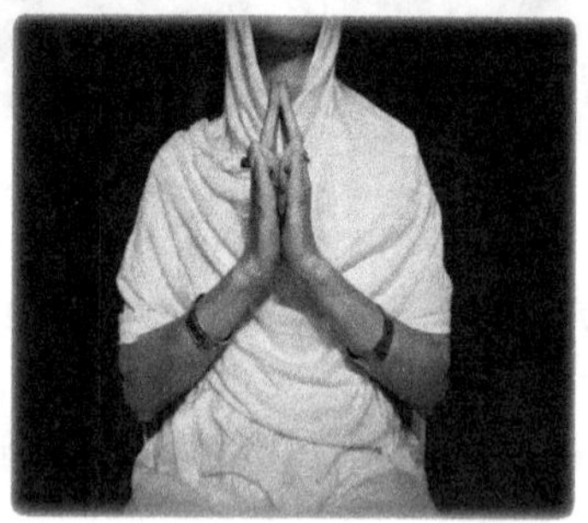

2nd picture, another angle 3rd and 4th Fingers Interlaced

Feeling sluggish, slow, outdated? Feel like your energy field is a leaky ship?

Be like the fox!

Internal

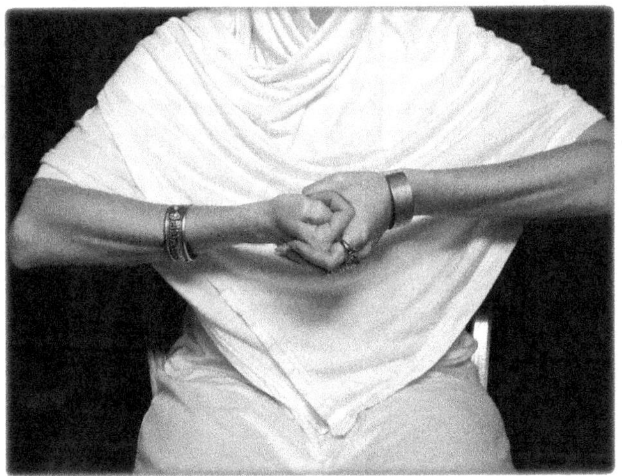

Thumb Inside Wrapped Fingers

Retreat, curling inwards. Taking a breather. Hibernating for the winter.

Have you been too active? Doing way too many things in the physical, overloading your system? Spreading to much time with other people, interacting with various forms of media?

Take a break.

External

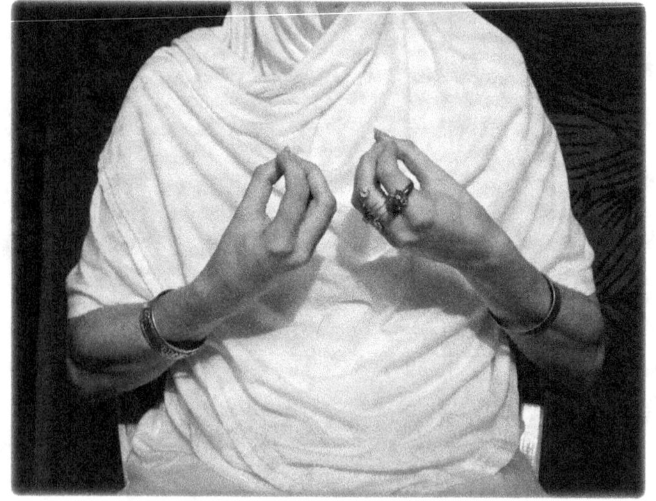

All Fingertips Touching Thumb

Buds in springtime. Unfurling forth, onwards and upwards.

Spread your wings out of your cocoon.

Reach out to those who need you. Understand your place in the greater scheme of things.

Unified Consciousness

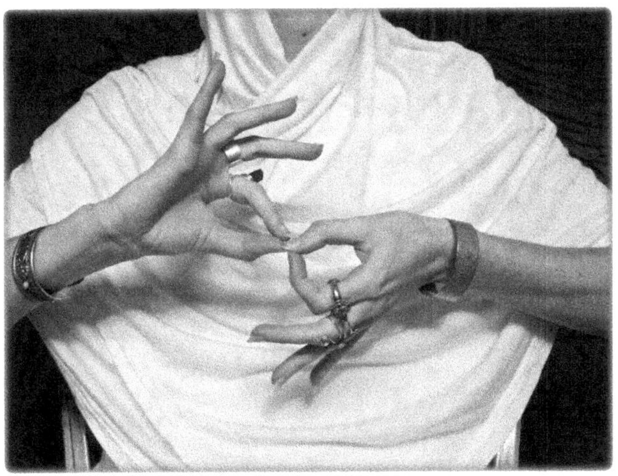

1st Finger and Thumb Touch, All Other Fingers Spread

When polarities are balanced within us, they cease to exist. Have you been thinking in extreme black and white lately? Swinging from one extreme thought and back again?

Piece back together your consciousness, parts of yourself over space and time. Reclaim lost bits of your unconscious like defragmentation of your energy field.

True Expression

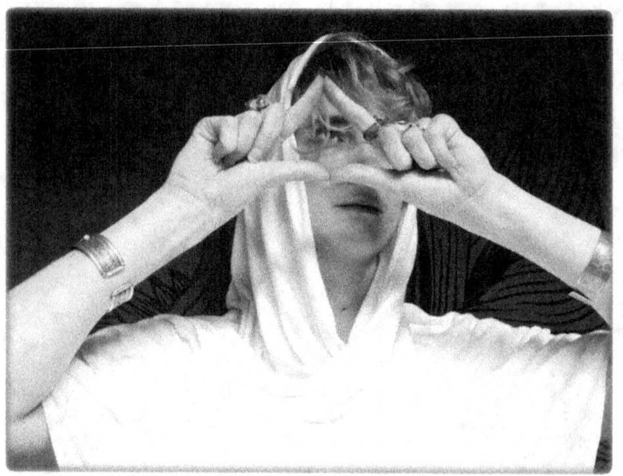

1st and Thumbs touch, All Other Fingers Curled In Tightly

What is your truth as a human expressing the eternal in the now?

What lies do you want to stop believing in? What kind of life do you really want to live?

Still unsure? Get sure!

What is your own personal brand of truth you must share with the world?

Action

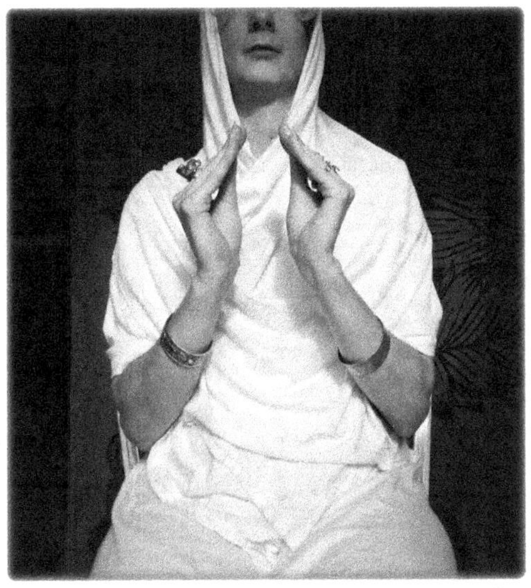

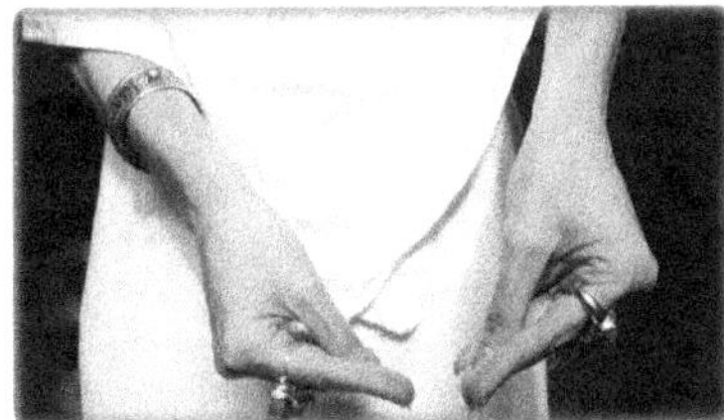

Thumbs Inbetween 1st and 2nd Fingers

Are there some things that you need to do but aren't doing them? Procrastination your middle name? Perhaps you have started something but things keep getting in the way, making more and more delays. Cultivate perseverance and get moving again!

The Spark

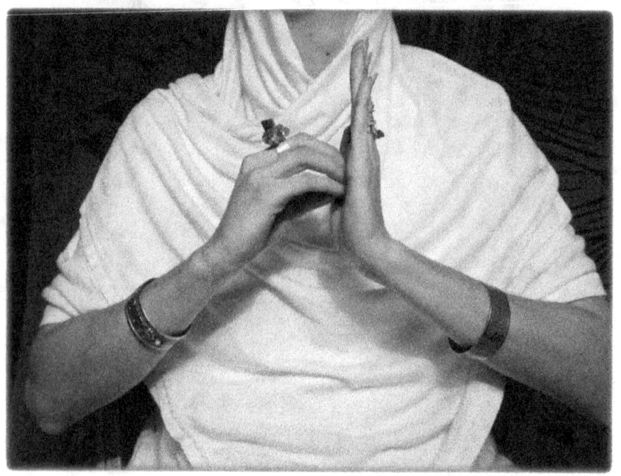

All Fingers Touching Thumb In Middle of Other Palm

Spontaneity. Release your writer's block.

Let your inner children fly free!

Stop overthinking and worrying about will or won't be.

Rewaken your Spark of Creation.

Fluid Movement

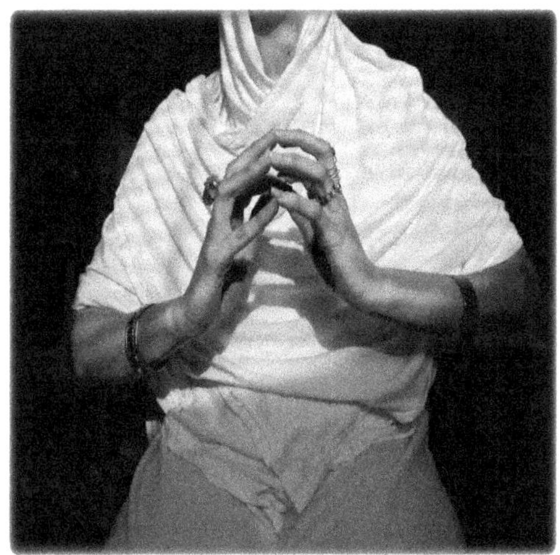

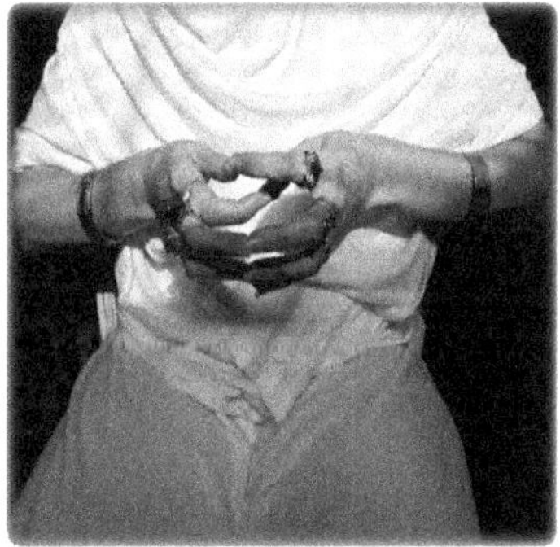

1st Finger to Thumb Reversed

Have you become rigid? Have you mind taken over your life? Do you spend too much time compartmentalizing your life and everyone in it? Do you spend way too much time looking at the tiny details, making more as you go along and not at the larger picture?

Make peace with the element of water, feeling your emotions and letting them go.

Manifested Goal

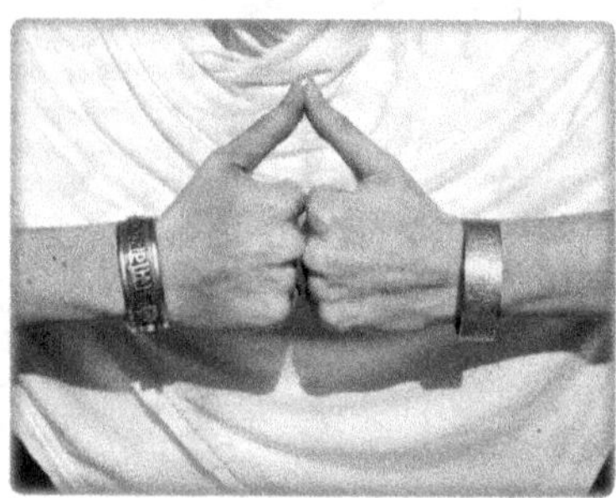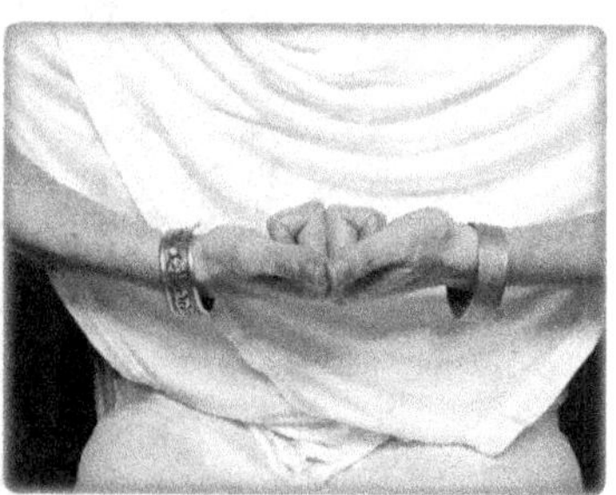

Thumb to Thumb, All Other Fingers Tightly Curled

Have you made intentions that you want to see manifested into the physical?

Perhaps you feel like your dreams need a boost of extra energy.

Intend the fulfillment of all your intended dreams, no compromises.

Integrity

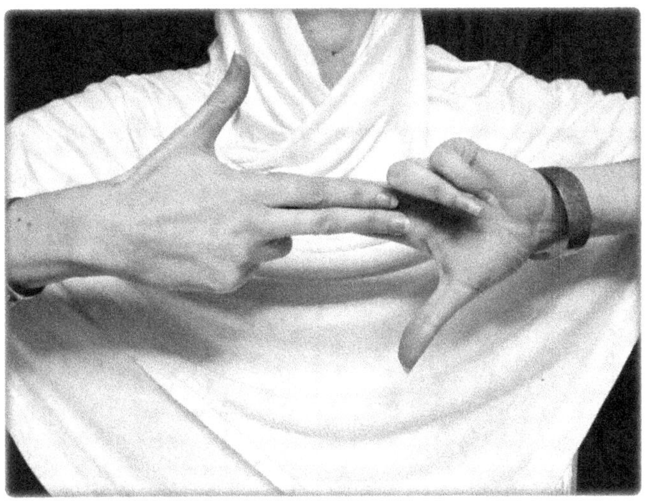

Underneath Finger Straight Against Upper Fingers

Do you sometimes do something when inside, you really want to be doing something else?

Are you two faced? Do you pretend? Do you fake it?

Are you afraid to stand in your truth and say what you really feel?

Are you afraid to show the world who you really are?

This is the perfect mudra!

Visioning

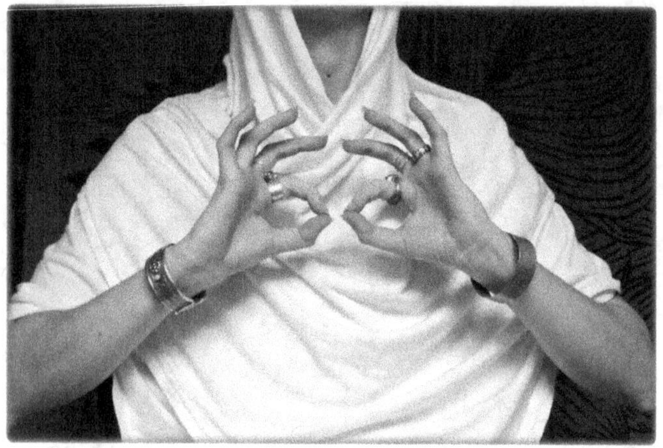

Receive a vision for your life. Open your intuitive channels. Go on a shamanic journey. Do you feel like you don't have a future? Feel dead inside? Feel like you have no purpose?

There's no need to continue feeling like that!

Activate your inner visionary.

The Dream

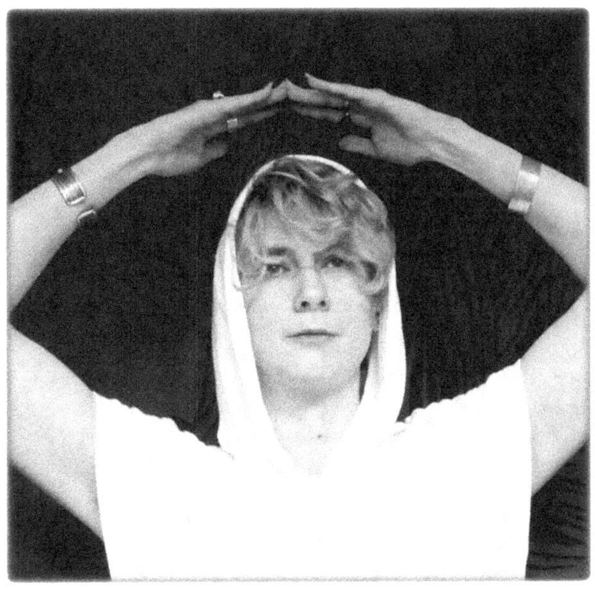

Middle Fingers Touch

Remember how to dreamweave. Deeply understand the nature of manifestation.

Be like spider, always taking care of your nest/web.

Always getting what you need and more. Learn how to receive and be the container.

Igniting Passions

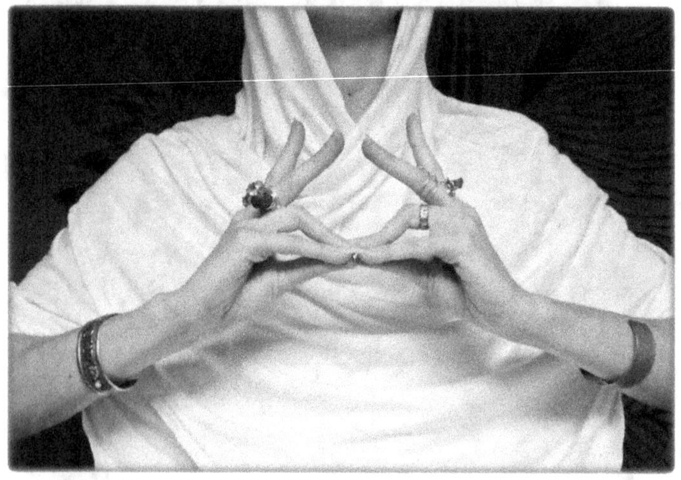

3rd 4th fingers to Thumbs

What is your passion? Do you feel like you have lost it?

As children, we express our passions without reserve. Receive this lost expression, infuse your life with passion and watch everything change around you.

Passion is the driving force that some might misinterpret as anger.

Also associated with the air element, sit with this mudra to make peace with this element.

Activating The Kundahlini
3 Movements

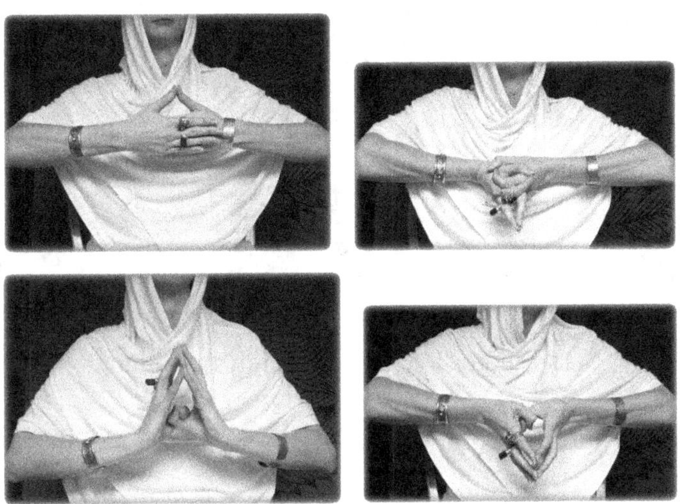

1st Picture – 1st Movement, Underneath hand flat against top hand
2nd Picture – 2nd Movement, 1st Finger and Thumb Touching, 2nd
Fingers Touch, Fingers Interlaced
3rd and 4th Picture – 3rd Movement, Thumbs Wrapped, Rest of
Fingers Touching

The Kundahlini is a very powerful energy at the base of your base.
Released, it can fuel your life and spiritual endeavors.

Learn how it feels to become like a volcano within.

Make peace with the fire element and your expression of sexuality.

Communion

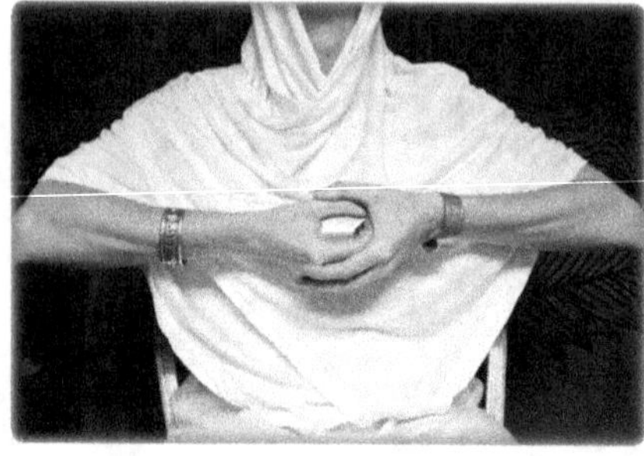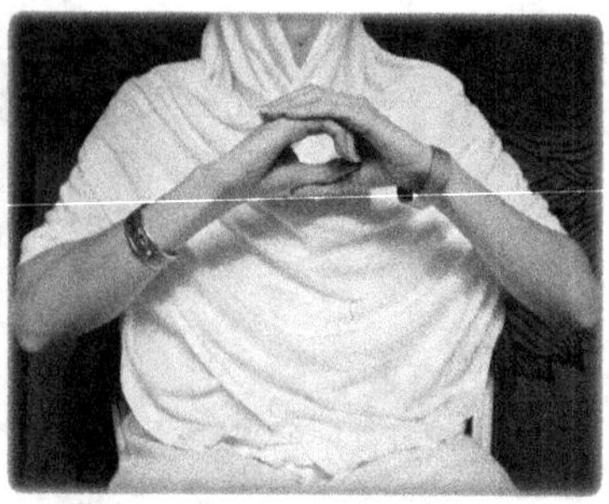

1st Finger and Thumb Lightly Touch

Want to learn how to communicate with the plants? With the animals?

With any consciousness on Earth?

Intend to bring forth translation movements within your field and enter another consciousness' creation in honor.

You will understand, and hear what you need to hear.

Communicate with feeling, beyond thought.

Sit in reverence and silence with other aspects of creation.

Dance Of Being

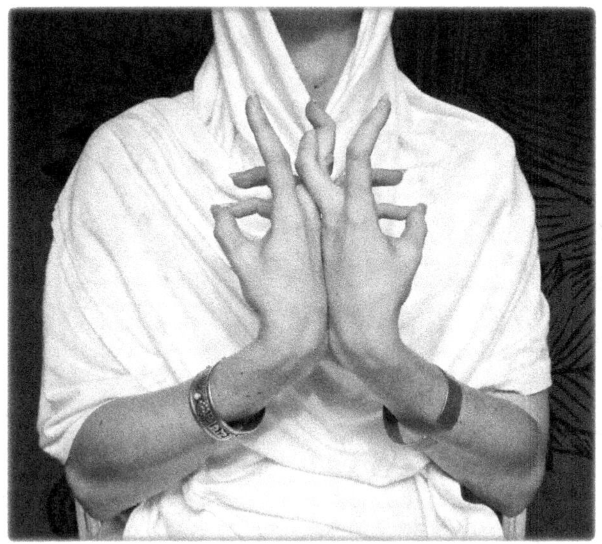

2nd Finger Wrapped, 4th Finger to Thumb

We dance.

Move in and out of time. Move in and out of experience. In and out of body after body. In and out of one solar system to the next, one way of perceiving to the next.

One set of limitations, thoughtforms to the next.

We dance.

Silence

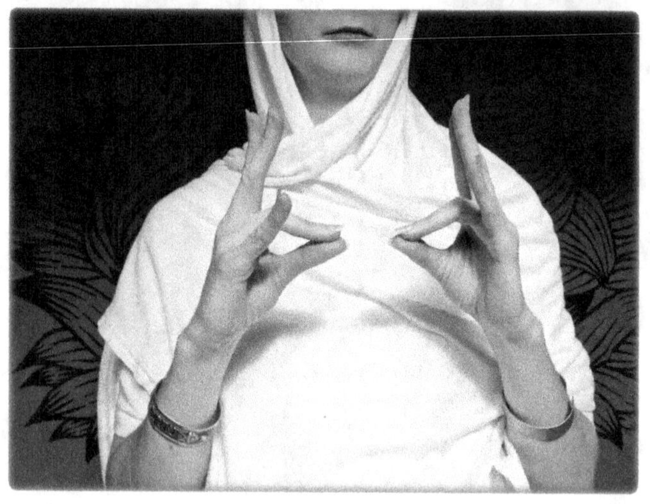

Middle Finger Pad to Thumb

Silence is …

The Everlasting AUM

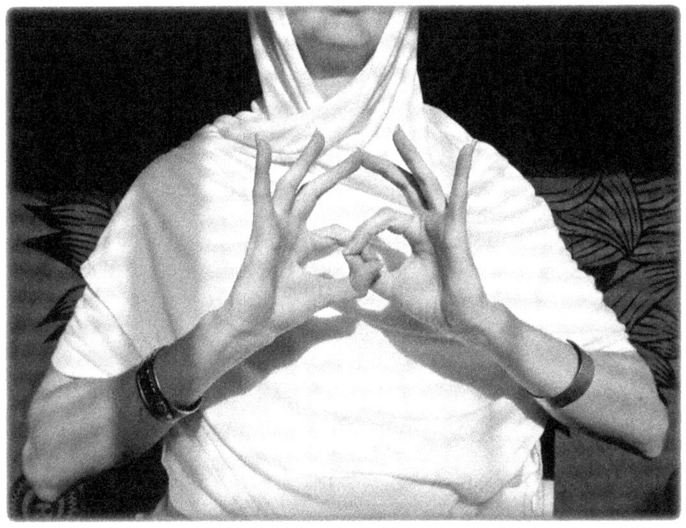

Middle Finger to Middle Finger, 1st Finger to Thumb, interlocked

As we move our timeless bodies into the eternal dreamtime of forever land, we remember to breathe our collected thoughts into a breathless prye and we sink into oblivion for a moment.

Remembering again who we really are

Who we really are

the eternal aum

REMEMBER

All movements are made to recognize the wholeness that already is.

Extras

Ancestral Recasting

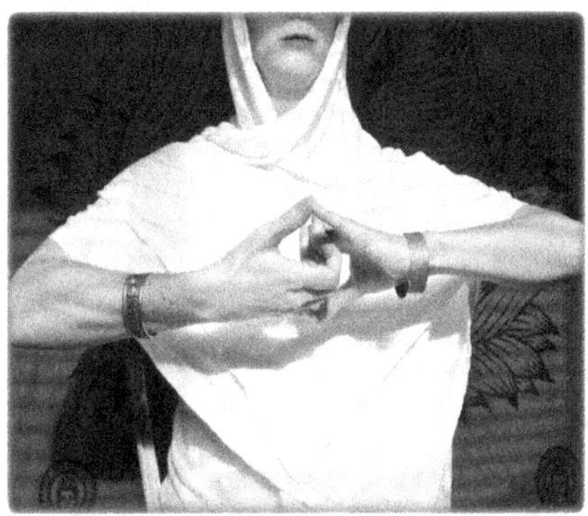

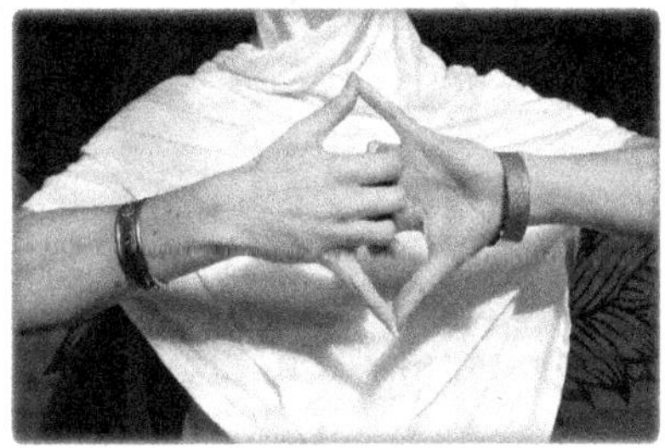

1st thru 3rd fingers bent, wrapped Thumb to 4th fingerpads

The Ancestors are always in the background. If we want to reclaim
their gifts into our life, we need to call them forward. This mudra is
for clarifying our ancestral lines and bringing forward the DNA and
associated gifts we want to embody in this lifetime.

Overwhelmed Heart

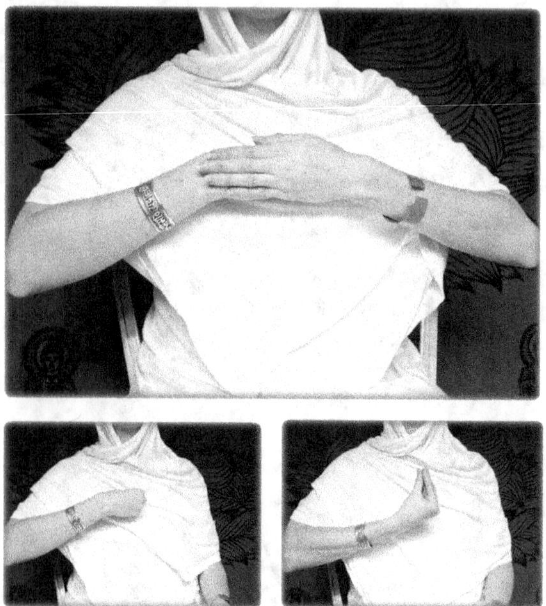

1st bottom picture – position of hand underneath top hand
2nd bottom picture – how fingers are held, all fingers tightly held to thumb

If you are prone to anxiety attacks and have a hard time coping with high levels of stress, this mudra can help you a lot.

This mudra helps you remember to breathe and that this too shall pass.

Great Series
Great Mother

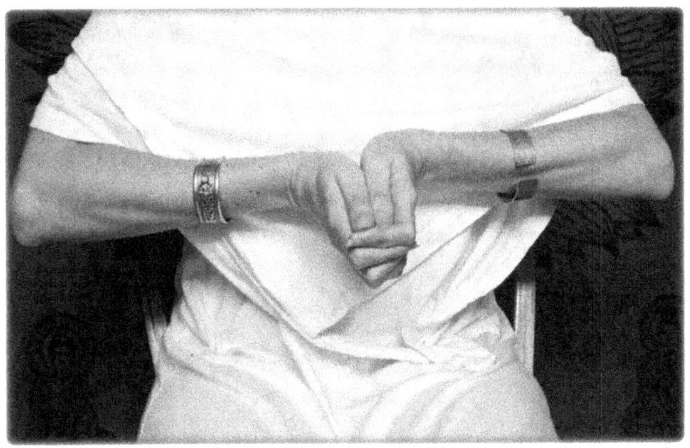

Inside fingers tightly curled inside

Sometimes we need to remember what deep nurturing is.

We recognize the so-called support and love we received from our parents is something we could hardly call either love or support, definitely not nurturing.

This mudra is perfect for becoming the parents we never had to ourselves, to understand and really feel deep love and safe nurturing.

Great Series
Great Reset

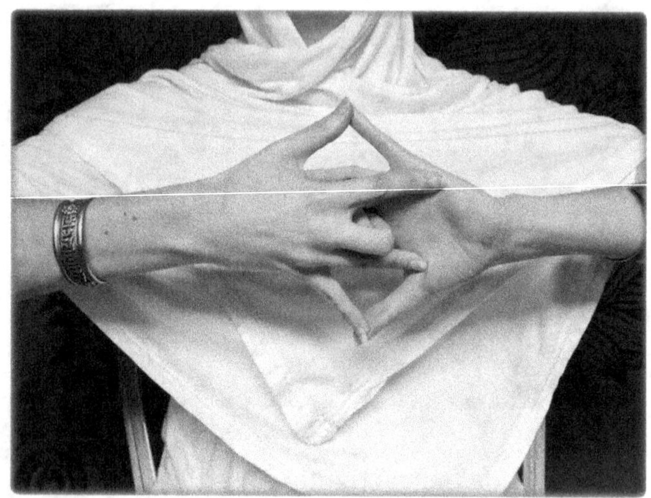

1st part of 2nd fingers bent, holding firmly
1st and 3rd fingers straight, resting on other hand Thumb to
4th fingerpads touch

I liken this mudra to the Titanic, not only turning around, but completely lifting off the sea bed and then sailing to the new old, brand new!

If you need a deep rebirth in your life, don't underestimate the power of this mudra.

Ignition Of Twin Heart Flame Within

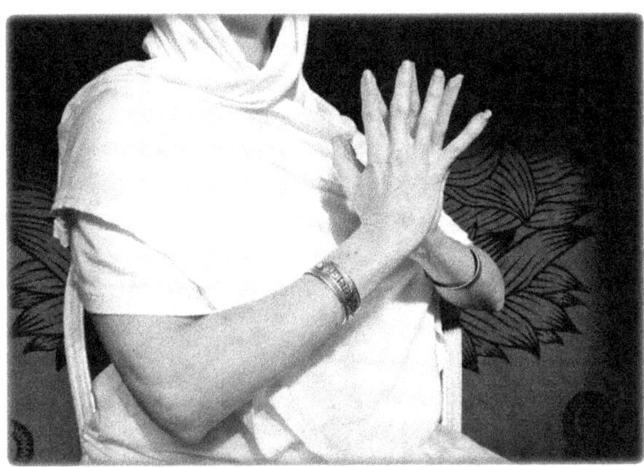

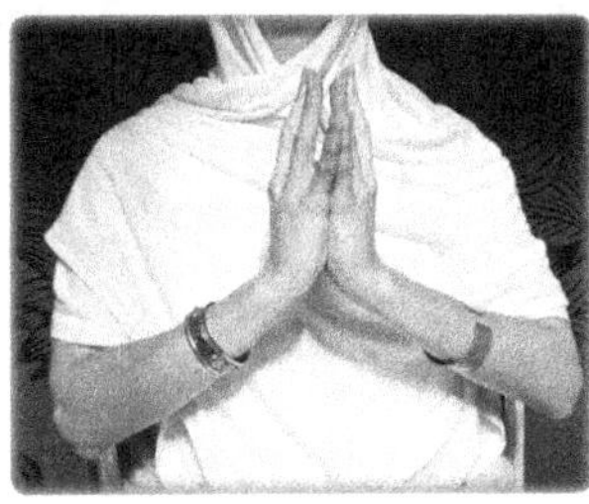

1st, 4th and Thumb Fingerpads Touch, Middle and 3rd Finger Free
Bottom of Hands Touch

Ignite the twin flame within! The twin flame is a special blessing for ultimate union and supreme grace to enter our lives. The union of our cosmic male and female of our universal heart within of the grandest order, this mudra brings about the perfect relationship with our Beloved, in divine timing and splendid beauty.

Lotus Petal Breath

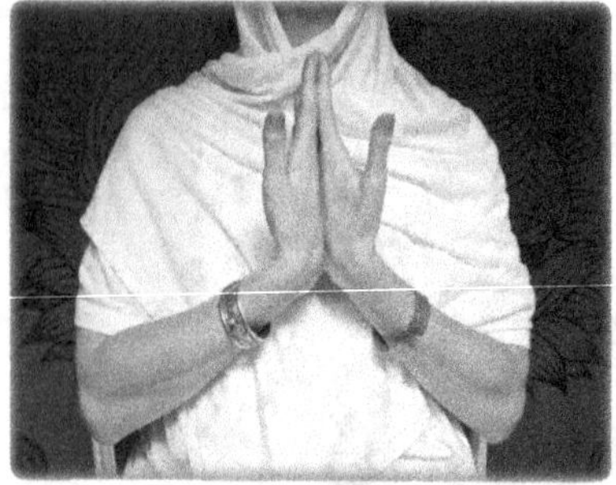 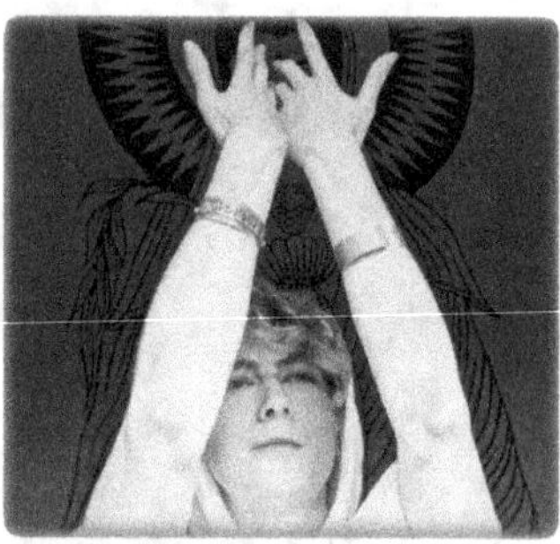

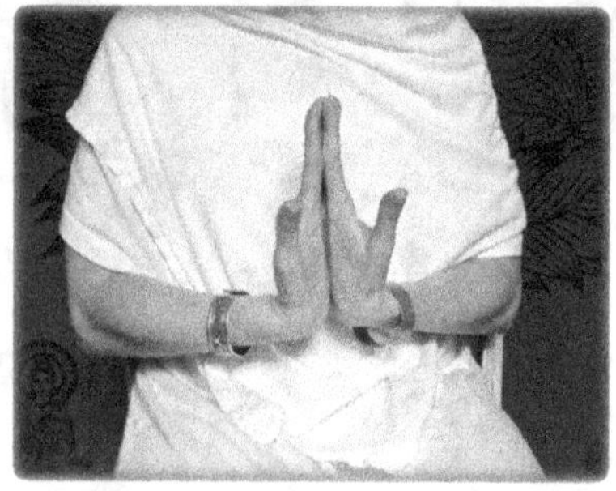

Start with your hands at your heart, moving up, keeping your breath in tune with the speed of your hands.

Reach up as high as you can and then bring back down in a circle, always keeping the backs of your hands as together as possible.

It doesn't matter when you breath in and out, just so long it's the same rhythm with your hands.

This movement mirrors the lotus growing from the swamp and blossoming forth, bringing gentleness and soft healing energy.

Eating The Essence

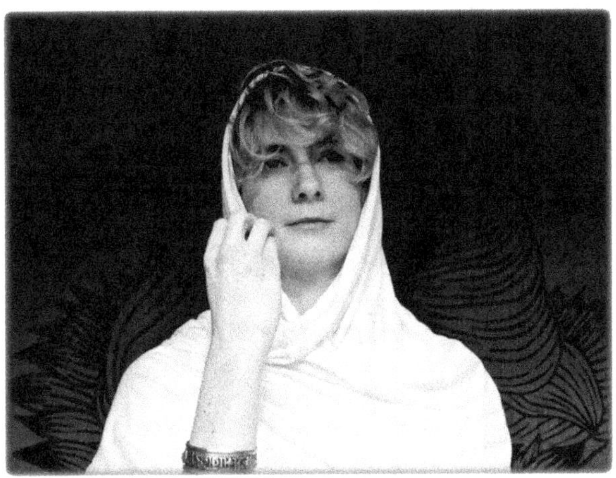

1-4th Fingertips Touch Thumb

Yogis have learned how to subsist on the air prana for thousands of years.

Forming the mudra and then bringing it to your mouth while imagining ingesting light and energy from the sun and beyond sustains your body in a new/old way.

Bring the mudra to your mouth as if you are eating.

Mudra
Healing

The Path To Recognizing The Truest Essence
Is Paved With Contemplation

Mudras are inherently silent and loud at the same time.

They move our energy bodies in new ways and in this we see how
our bodies and energy fields associated are completely interrelated.
We may silently do them or add mantra to the moment, either way,
it is done with intention, purpose in our heart and contemplation.

We place our focus towards the eternal and what we are given in
return in boundlessness wrapped in silence, feeling beyond words
and a peace in our hearts that is everlasting.

Mudra can help us get there, in a gentle, non-forcing but poignant
way.

Mudra is a time tested, mother approved way to really express the
feeling you have always been. Peace, wellness, wholeness. These are
the basis tenants, rights and expression of everything creational
aspect within the whole. If you are feeling anything other than this,
then that means you are living in a lie, or multiple lies that have
compounded.

The greater disease and un-ease in your life, the greater the lie you
have agreed with live with.

When we have forgotten, we mudra to remember who we are really
are. We focus on the truth of our timelessness and drop back into
the rhythm, the sound, the movement of all that is, of the eternal.
The natural world order.

The act of doing mudra is so simple and yet so effective. It efficiently calls to us just what we need, in the moment we need it. We come back into the movement to realize just what we need to realize. We return to our true selves, our true expression.
Miracles occur, shifts in perception happen. Just when we think we will be stuck in some kind of mind loop, we do a mudra and everything is lifted.

Mudra is a blessing from the eternal realm unto the physical to reap the benefits of. To help us, to guide and to lighten our way home, to mukti, moksha, getting off the wheel of karma, cause and effect.

To the ultimate presence that is who we are truly.

Get Creative!

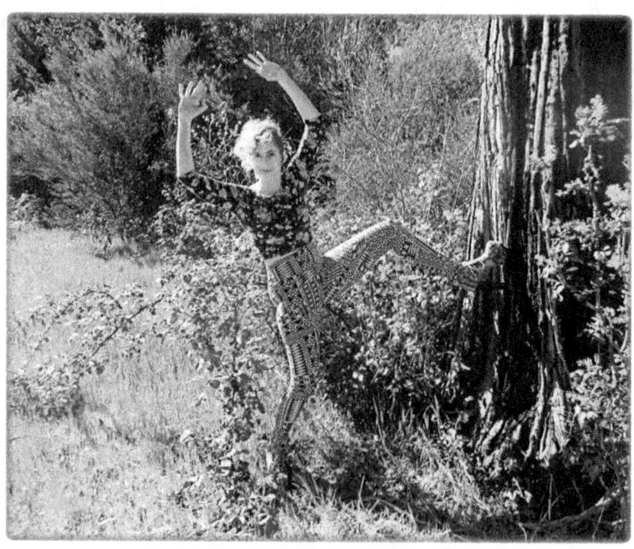

So, you might have this idea, per various images you have seen that mudra is only to be done at certain times. You've seen the image of the mediator sitting, eyes closed, classic yoga pose. We do 'yoga' for an hour or so, and then go back to 'whatever we were doing before.'

I want to let you know you can mudra whenever, why ever … If doesn't have to look and be all 'traditional,' this is experiential. It doesn't need to be somber all the time. You don't even have to do mudra for yourself, you can do it for other people!

It doesn't always have to be a long ritual, they can be done for short periods of time, on the go.

Let's incorporate mudra into your daily life while you make your whole existence be your yoga.

The Blessing Way

Here are some different ways to use mudra to bless yourself, bless the elements and bless other people!

Sleeping and Waking with Mudra

Before going to sleep, pick out the mudra or mudra sequence you would like to do. Make it your evening meditation. Make it as long or as short as you feel you need.

For in the morning, upon waking but before opening your eyes, move your hands and fingers into position without looking, just feeling and sinking in.

Feel the peace and let this carry you throughout the rest of the day or the night!

Mudra with Mineral and Herb

If you are a rock person, you can sit or lay down and meditate with your favorite crystal (or many) while holding the mudra.

You can place the crystal on your body or you can put it inside the mudra!

You can also do this with herbs. There are so many herbs that are beneficial to our wellbeing. Either instead of or while ingesting the herb, you could also hold it in your hand while doing the mudra.

This way, you could commune and communicate with the consciousness of the Herb to bring different blessings into your life.

Eating With Mudra Food Blessing

Before eating, you could hold the food with a particular mudra in order to bless the food with the vibration the mudra anchors.

Direct blessings, internally!

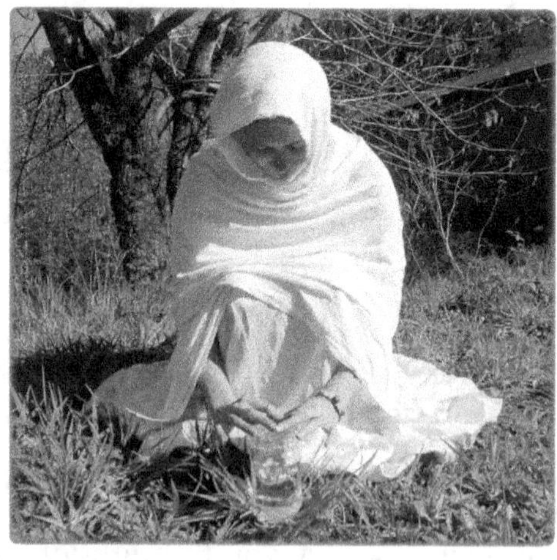

Drinking With Mudra
Water Blessing

Perhaps you've heard of Dr Emoto and blessing water with good thoughts? Similar instance, just with mudra AND good thought combined.

To change the quality of the water and bring the blessings deeper into your life, hold the mudra next to the glass filled with water or position the glass inbetween your hands.

Think of whatever qualities you want the water to be infused with, focus on this for a few minutes. Drink to your blossoming awareness!

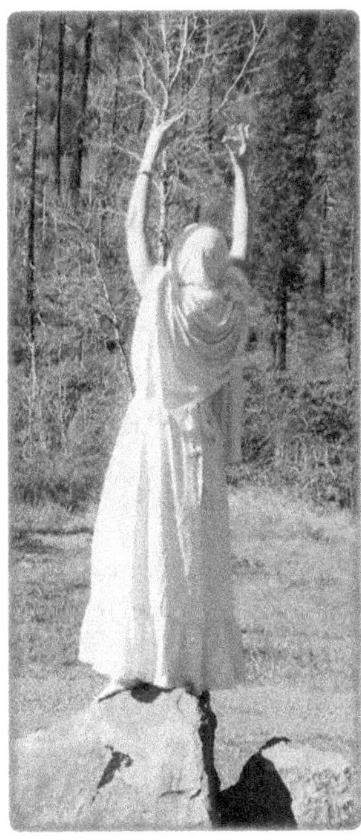

Earth + Garden Blessing

Plants naturally respond to our thoughts, feelings and energy flow. If you have a garden, you can bless it naturally with your presence. Sitting down and meditating in gardens is something the Ancestors have done since the beginning of Time.
You can do whatever mudra you feel best and then intend that the blessings are sent to the Earth and the Plants equally, infusing your garden with love.

And when you eat of the fruit of your garden, the love returns full force!

Energy Healing In Person or Long Distance
Human Blessing

If you already do some kind of energy healing practice then this will be like second nature. If not, it's always fun to try!

Anyone can do it, it doesn't take a master or any special kind of training or certificate. All that it requires is focus and everybody can do that!

For long distance, set some time aside to get very quiet and clear, make sure you are in a space where you will not be easily distracted. Think of the person in your mind who needs the healing while holding the mudra. Imagine this person or people openly receiving this energy that you are sending them.

For in person, simply form the mudra with your hands and place your hands near or on the person where you feel their energy body needs it the most.

Mudra Meditation

While doing mudra, it can fun be to play with the meditation time.

You can incorporate color healing for your aura. You can move through every color of the rainbow, you can do the whole rainbow at once. Imagine it swirling through your field.

You can also try metallic essences such as gold, silver, cooper and see how that feels.

Another thing you can try is creating an image in your mind that you really love. Flying through the Universe, a beautiful forest or field, inside a volcano, who knows. Someplace that is very close to your heart, very fulfilling and healing to experience.

The last suggestion involves intentions. If you have a intention that is very important to you, just simply repeat that in your head like a modern day mantra as long as you hold the mudra.

Talk about keeping your mind focused!

Mudra Yoga

Perhaps you already have s strong yoga practice. You can incorporate mudra into your poses that don't directly involve your hands, like the warrior and tree stance.

See how different it feels with mudra and what dimension it adds to your practice. You might be pleasantly surprised!

Dancing With Mudra

If you like to dance, try adding mudra to your dance. Mudra is not stagnant, even tho you do hold your fingers and hands together in a certain way. Some people receive more healing energy from moving instead of sitting still. If you are one of those people, then you could benefit greatly from doing this.

In Conclusion

I hope this book brings many blessings into your life.

The mudra were a gift to me from the Ancestors, including Agastya, a maharishi from Ancient India who has also been a friend and provided nonphysical support during childhood until high school days, then lost connection but returned while taking a Yoga Teacher Training course.

I am so happy to be able to share them with everyone!

Namaste.
the stillness within me witnesses the stillness within you

may you realize the infinite blessing that you are!

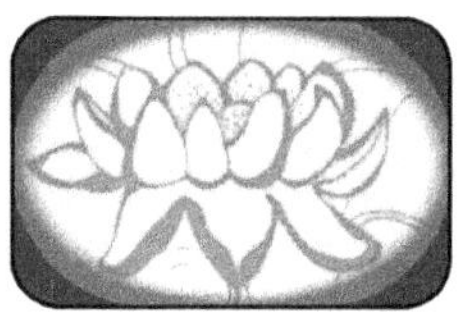

*the limitless eternal changeless
Self is You!*